GLUTEN FREE
IN 48 HOURS

The Beginner's Guide to a Gluten Free Life

By Tom Harris

www.glutify.co.uk

Gluten Free In 48 Hours
Copyright and Disclaimer

Have you been diagnosed with the following conditions?

- Coeliac Disease

- Gluten Intolerance

Or are you just deciding to go gluten free?

Are you looking to go gluten free as fast as possible? Do you feel overwhelmed and unsure how to get started? You might be wondering how on earth to cut gluten out of your life.

Well you have picked up the right guide. This book answers all these questions.

Unlike many of the books you will find on Amazon, this book isn't a textbook guide on the science behind going gluten free. It also isn't stuffed with loads of complicated recipes you would see on a cooking program. This is a simple, practical book designed to help you get gluten free as quickly as possible.

If you are going to stick to a new lifestyle then you need a plan that is easy to follow. We are all busy people and you do not have time to be scouring the internet for answers.

What you need is a step by step plan that helps you get started. And helps you understand where to start and what you need to prioritise first.

This book is here to help you:

- Go gluten free fast! (it can be done in 48 hours)

- Make your kitchen safe

- Learn where to buy gluten free products

- Discover meals you can prepare to get started

- Avoid mistakes beginners make

Why you should remove gluten fast!

If you have been diagnosed with coeliac disease then it is very important you take action today.

Do not continue to eat gluten!

Eating gluten will do permanent damage to your intestines. You only get one set of intestines to last you a lifetime. The doctors can't replace this part of your body. Once they're shot to bits, that's it - you'll either be eating through a tube or pooping into a bag for the rest of your days.

I am not here to scare you into action but continued abuse has been linked to more serious diseases. You have a higher risk of developing...

- Malnutrition

- Dermatitis Herpetiformis

- Thyroid Disease

- Diabetes

- Cancer

And even if you are only gluten sensitive, do you really want to live with pain, discomfort and fatigue?

The benefits of going gluten free

Apart from avoiding the increased risk of developing further diseases, there are many reasons why you should go gluten free.

You might have been battling symptoms of coeliac for months or even years before being diagnosed. You could have years of damage that needs to be addressed.

Imagine a life where you are no longer plagued with stomach pains. Where you do not live in constant pain.

One of my friends said living with coeliac is like waking up as a 90 year old every day.

No one wants to feel like that, do they?

Eliminate gluten in 48 hours

My promise to you is that this book will help you get started quickly.

You can go gluten free in 48 hours.

You will start to see an improvement in your symptoms.

It will take away your overwhelming feeling of having so much to change because you get a step by step process to follow.

Who am I?

My name is Tom Harris. You might be surprised to hear this but I am not coeliac and I do not have intolerance to gluten.

What I do have though are many friends that can't eat gluten.

They have been through the same journey you are about to make.

They couldn't imagine life without bread or pizza.

How am I qualified to teach people how to go gluten free?

I helped my friends when they had no one to turn to. When it feels like no one understands their condition. When they felt like the only person in the world suffering from this disease.

I have been doing this for years. In the process it has made me quite the expert. This led to me starting up Glutify™ which aims to help those who want to live a gluten free life.

I have firsthand experience helping others get started. I learned from scratch. I was in the same place you are now. I knew nothing.

I chose to learn. I didn't want to be another one of those friends that thinks 'just a little biscuit won't hurt.'

I excel at breaking things down into simple to follow processes. That is what I have done with this book. Think of this book as one large checklist of everything I learned and now pass along to you.

This book is everything my coeliac friends wished they had when they first started.

I hope the advice in this book helps you like it already has others.

CONTENTS

Dame Kelly Holmes returned from the 2004 Olympics a gold medal winner.

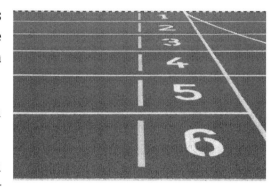

But it wasn't all plain sailing.

Kelly suffered from clinical depression. It took a huge amount of mental energy for her to stay on track.

Olympians must prepare every aspect of their life, their food and their routine to win. Injuries can derail their progress. They work with coaches who support and guide them in the right direction. They must be prepared to make major life decisions and sacrifices.

Kelly didn't wake up a gold medal winner. It took years of preparation and the right mindset to win.

Like an Olympian, you are making a major life change too.

It takes the same level of preparation to live a gluten free life.
You have to plan ahead for everything. You have to prepare every meal from scratch. Scrutinise everything you do and eat.

If you eat gluten it can derail your progress, set back your healing. You have dietitians, doctors and online communities to support and guide you.

That is why this book exists. It was created to help you win.

Adopt an Olympian mindset

If there is one mindset you must adopt quickly, it is devotion to relentless preparation.

- Preparing your meals in advance

- Preparing your trips to the supermarket

- Preparing your trips out to restaurants

- Preparing your ingredients to ensure they are safe

- Preparing your trips to visit friends and family

- Preparing your kitchen surfaces

The list is endless. If you are not prepared you will get caught off guard. You will make mistakes and derail your progress.

Your Free Gift

I created this cheat sheet (**www.glutify.co.uk/gluten-free-cheatsheet**) to help you stay prepared and gluten free.

Download it before you begin and use it alongside this book. It will give you the opportunity to sign up for my newsletter, and receive daily support emails and extra tips to help you get started.

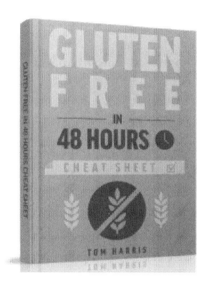

www.glutify.co.uk/gluten-free-cheatsheet

CHAPTER 1:

Found Out you Can't Eat Gluten? Do This First

Day 1 Tips

You can't start to remove gluten fast until you fully understand what condition you have. If you haven't officially been diagnosed by a doctor via a blood test or biopsy then I recommend doing this before reading the rest of this book.

What to do when you are struggling to understand your condition

If you are at this stage and you do not understand your condition fully, then visit our website at **www.glutify.co.uk/understanding-your-condition** and download your free bonus guide.

This resource will help you understand what stage you are at with your diagnosis. What you could *potentially* be suffering from and how to get officially diagnosed.

Why you should get diagnosed

If you don't get diagnosed before you remove gluten from your diet, you will never get properly diagnosed. Doctors need to see how your body reacts to gluten. You do not want to go gluten free and then find you need to revert back for proper tests.

It will also make it easier to inform other people of your condition when you have an official diagnosis. Trust me. You will be explaining to a lot of people from now on why you can't eat toast!

CHAPTER 2:

The Gluten Free Escape Plan

Day 1 Tips

Right, so you are officially diagnosed as coeliac or with a gluten intolerance. Let's get started.

This book aims to improve your symptoms in the first 48 hours. The end goal is to get gluten out of your system. You want to ensure your gut goes into healing mode to avoid any long term health effects as we discussed earlier.

It takes time for gluten to leave your system

How long does it actually take? That varies from person to person.

In your first 48 hours of going gluten free, you should start seeing improvements to your symptoms. In most cases gluten won't fully leave your system for 3 full months. This will only happen if you follow a strict gluten free diet.

Once you get rid of the gluten in your system you may still experience symptoms from the damage already caused to your intestines. Some people have symptoms for years.

How to know when gluten starts leaving your system

How soon you notice the benefits of gluten leaving your system depends on your gluten sensitivity level.

Symptoms like brain fog, fatigue and swelling have been known to subside substantially in the first 48 hours. Bowel symptoms should also start to improve after a couple of days.

How to speed up the healing process in 3 steps

If you want speed up the time it takes to heal your gut, you need to take the following into account:

1. Don't cheat! Just a bite won't hurt will it? It most certainly will. Every time you ingest gluten you slow down your body's healing process. One bite of gluten could set you back a couple of weeks or even start your healing process over from the beginning.

Do not give in to the cookie. Do not eat the cookie!

2. Drink more water. We do not get enough water in our standard diets, and many people in the world are chronically dehydrated. If you want to improve detoxification then improve your hydration.

The recommended amount of water you should drink has always been debated but some guidelines to get you started are:

1. Women = 2 litres a day (8 cups)

2. Men = 3 litres a day (13 cups)

3. Eat fruits and vegetables. Along with drinking more of water, you should eat lots of fruits and vegetables. This will improve your bowel transit time—the time it takes food to travel through your digestive tract—and help remove gluten from your body. Having one or two bowel movements each day is a sign of a healthy gut.

Disclaimer: Despite doing all of the above, you may not be able to speed up the healing process. Existing health conditions, like kidney and liver problems, may cause your healing to progress slowly. Your genetics or your sensitivity to gluten can also affect healing speed. Keep your head up in these situations—all you can do is your best.

Let's move onto what causes these symptoms—gluten.

There is a war going on in your stomach

Right now there is a war raging in your gut between your immune system and gluten.

It's time to stop the enemy. Let's start with what NOT to eat, and learn what you need to stay clear of going forwards. Gluten is often hidden in many everyday items so we'll learn which ones to avoid.

Grains are gluten in its natural form so you need to ensure you avoid the following ingredients:

- Barley, including barley malt
- Bran
- Bulgur
- Farina
- Wheat
- Kamut
- Orzo
- Semolina
- Spelt

You could spend ages searching for products containing these ingredients. The problem with this list is that it doesn't really narrow down your search for what foods you can or can't eat.

In the next chapter we will discuss what foods you should be avoiding, so you can get started quickly.

CHAPTER 3:

How to Eliminate Gluten from your Kitchen

Day 1 Tips

You know what gluten-filled foods to look out for. Now it's time to head to the kitchen and remove items containing those ingredients.

Your aim by the end of your first day is to remove every bit of gluten from your kitchen.

To prevent food waste, collect everything together and either give it to a friend or donate it to your local food bank. If you live in the UK check out The Trussell Trust to donate your food. If you are from the US then pay a visit to your local Food Bank.

It is important at this stage to completely eliminate gluten from your kitchen. Let's look at the key products you need to remove.

7 products you need to remove from your kitchen

Let's start with the fridge and food cupboards. If yours are like mine, they are probably due for a good cleaning anyway! This is going to take a couple of hours. Make sure you clear everything with any hint of gluten out before moving on.

1. Jars and condiments. Every jar and container will need to be inspected, especially if they have been opened. If something is in a jar you should stop using it to avoid any contamination that may have been caused by cutlery. Can you imagine a knife that has been used to spread peanut butter onto toast? Once it goes back into the jar you have cross contamination from the bread. A number of products in open containers are gluten free but I recommend replacing them to avoid previous incidents of contamination.

Types of products to look out for: honey, peanut butter, ketchup, jam, marmalade, mustard.

2.   Baking ingredients. Flour is the obvious one here as it contains gluten but what about the other ingredients you bake with? How can you be sure that you haven't contaminated them with flour? Before you run off to replace all of your cooking ingredients, wait until you have time to think about and plan cooking gluten free meals. There are many new ingredients you will need in the future.

Types of products to look out for: caster sugar, salt, yeast, olive oil.

3. Baked goods. Baked goods are probably the easiest to spot and the biggest change to your diet. Unless it is certified as gluten free you are going to be giving away every baked item in your home. I would particularly highlight croutons as something to watch out for. These sneak into all sorts of meals (prepared salads, soups etc).

Types of products to look out for: pastries, dough, muffins, tortillas, bread, breadcrumbs, cakes, cookies, croutons.

4. Pasta and noodles. Avoid pasta and noodles—they are made from wheat. Don't get caught out by egg noodles, these also contain gluten.

Types of products to look out for: macaroni, spaghetti, penne, fusilli, noodles, egg noodles.

5. Cereals. Most cereals are made from wheat, rye or barley and if they are not they are most likely processed in a factory with these ingredients. Always check the label first. Watch out for oats and granola as even though these do not contain wheat, they are generally processed with products that are!

If you are really sensitive to Gluten do not touch oats or granola at all. I have known people with high gluten sensitivities to have reactions to oats that were certified gluten free.

Types of products to look out for: bran, mainstream cereal brands.

6. Meat, fish, and poultry. All meat is naturally gluten free until it is breaded, floured, fried or has sauces added. You should also avoid processed meats. Many of these have flavours added, which could contain gluten.

Types of products to look out for: fried chicken, breaded fish, sausages.

7. Canned and processed foods. Stay clear of canned processed meats as they normally have flour added to improve their texture. Similarly, stay clear of most canned products and processed meats unless labeled gluten free. They will usually have gluten-filled sauces or other nasties hidden to improve their quality.

Types of products to look out for: canned vegetables, canned pasta, canned soups, hot dogs, deli and luncheon meats.

All done? Then it's time to have a look at what equipment you have in your kitchen.

10 Items in your kitchen you need to make safe

It's not only food you need to watch out for in the war against gluten. You are going to have to scrutinise every piece of kitchen equipment.

1. **Toaster.** The toaster is the most dangerous piece of equipment in your kitchen. This is because it comes into direct contact with gluten, as in toast. You cannot clean your toaster and make it safe. You need to buy a new toaster and mark it off limits to everyone attempting to put non gluten free bread in it. You should also put it in a safe cupboard when you are done with it. You do not want crumbs falling into it when you are not using it.

2. **Oven.** You might think that your oven should be fairly safe. It might be, but I wouldn't take any risks. You should clean out your oven from top to toe. Get into all the little crevices with warm soapy water. If it has a little drip tray underneath, ensure you clean it out. Clean all the metal shelves that it comes with too.

You can never be too sure what your fan assisted oven might blow onto your food.

3. **Grill.** Get your own grill to cook meat. It will give you peace of mind and you will be able to segregate it from those in your household that might cook breaded meats or other gluten containing products. Like the toaster, store it in a cupboard or place that will be safe from contamination.

Little scratches and crevices on your grill can conceal gluten which can then sneak into your food.

4. **Fridge.** Once you have emptied your fridge of all those risky contaminants, wash it out with warm soapy water. If you will be sharing your fridge with someone else, make sure that you put all your stuff on the top shelf. You want to avoid gluten falling onto your food.

Ensure that all your products are labeled. You might even want to get some large plastic containers to keep your food in if you are very sensitive to gluten.

5. **Kitchen counters.** It would be such a shame to go through all the trouble of removing gluten then get caught out when you prepare your foods. Trust me a lot of people do. Always wash your preparation area down with hot soapy water before you prepare any food. You never know what crumbs could be lingering from the last person that used your kitchen.

6. **Dining table.** This might not be in your kitchen but it is important that you don't miss it. You do not want to go to great lengths trying to make your kitchen safe only to contaminate your food at the table. It is important to clean the surfaces where you eat. You don't want any loose crumbs from breakfast making their way into your food!

Let's now look at dishes and utensils. I would personally replace all of them so you can be sure you are not contaminating yourself without realising it.

7. **Plastic bowls and utensils.** You should remove and replace your plastic bowls and utensils. These scratch easily which allows gluten to catch in the scratch and unsuspectingly creep into your meals. You shouldn't prepare any gluten free meals with plastic utensils unless they are solely for gluten free use.

8. **Non-stick pots and pans.** Just like plastic, non-stick pots and pans can harbor gluten because they scratch easily. Cast-iron is important to watch out for because it is porous and can hide gluten. Pots and pans made from stainless steel or solid aluminum should be okay to reuse.

You will just need to wash them between gluten and gluten free use.

9. **Wooden bowls, chopping boards, and utensils.** Wooden items have the same challenges as plastic items. They can scratch easily and are also porous. That spells double trouble, so replace them before use.

10. **Colanders.** This is a sneaky one. You will be surprised what is hiding in all those little holes! If you plan on using a colander, get a new one.

How to replace your dishes and utensils

You may notice from the previous list that you won't have much left in terms of dishes and utensils. You have given most of them away!

Replace your equipment with glass and metal that isn't cast iron or non-stick. If you want to avoid any risk of contamination, invest in some surgical stainless steel cookware. This is non-porous and won't bleed into your food. The price is well worth it, as you get what you pay for.

If you don't plan on sharing your equipment with the family then you can use any type you want but make sure you label them for gluten free use only.

In the next section I will show you how to get started with food and equipment labels.

8 great ways to segregate in the kitchen

1. **Labels.** You should label every gluten free product in your kitchen. You could invest in a label machine but let's start with something simple. Just get some white sticky labels and a marker. I find that postage labels are the best for this. You can make the words GLUTEN FREE stand out nicely on them.

2. **Designated places.** There is no point labelling your products only for them to be contaminated by something containing gluten. Make sure you store all your refrigerated products on the top shelf in the fridge. You will also want a cupboard that is just for your food and toaster.

3. **Toaster bags.** If you are on the move or staying away from home then toaster bags are a must. They are protective bags that are toaster safe and prevent all the little gluten breadcrumbs contaminating your bread. These bags can be used over and over again.

4. **Plastic bottles of condiments.** Try to avoid buying products in glass jars. You will be tempted to use spoons to get the contents out, which will increase your risk of contamination. Get condiments in plastic containers, the 'squeezy' ones, so you can squeeze the contents out without any risk.

5. **Colour coding.** If you really want to improve segregation, think about buying coloured equipment in different colour sets. Kitchen equipment is available for purchase in most colours. Just choose the colours you want to designate as gluten safe versus unsafe and make sure they are contrasting colours like blue and red. You will never mix up your utensils again!

6. **Wash up separately.** You might think that your sink is safe because it is clean. Well you would be wrong. You can easily become contaminated by gluten in a shared kitchen. The sponge and the kitchen towel you use may harbour gluten from previous use.

Colour code your sponges and towels and ensure they are kept apart. If in doubt then throw away the sponge and get a new one.

Don't get contaminated at the last hurdle.

7. **Prepare gluten free meals first.** If you share a household with others, there's a good chance you are preparing both gluten and gluten free meals. And you will probably be making these at similar times. Always make sure you prepare your gluten free meals first. It will reduce the risk of contamination and minimize mistakes. It's easy to get confused when it's all systems go in the kitchen. It only takes one wrong spatula in your food to mess up your meal.

8. **If in doubt, go without.** This applies to anything in your new diet. If you think that something contains gluten or has been contaminated then you shouldn't risk it. *Do not take the risk.* If you doubt something is gluten free then you are most likely right. Will it be worth the days of recovery if you do risk it?

Day 1 summary

We have reached the end of day 1. At this point you should have:

- A basic understanding of what foods you are trying to avoid.

- Removed unsafe products from your kitchen.

- Set up your kitchen so it is safe to store and prepare food gluten free.

It's time to get some sleep. Tomorrow you will be filling your life with gluten free foods.

CHAPTER 4:

Keep it Simple and Stick to your Diet

Day 2 Tips

You don't need fancy recipes to start eating gluten free. You need a simple formula to follow, and easy guidelines like the ones below.

Gluten appears in almost anything that has been processed by people. The less processing involved, the less chance there is of gluten.

Try to eat foods in their most natural form

What does this actually mean? Well, you want to eat foods that haven't been processed.

For example a chicken breast has been cut from a chicken but that is the only process involved so it is most likely gluten free. Take it to the next level with a breaded chicken breast. This has been processed further with breadcrumbs. It now definitely contains gluten.

Keep it simple

It is important at this stage not to overcomplicate your diet. If you do, you won't stick to it.

I could provide countless recipes in this book but do you really have the time to cook for 2 or 3 hours a day, following them to the letter? I doubt you do. Remember to keep things as simple as possible. There is a lot to take in.

Follow the simple guidelines below. You can mix and match these foods to create different meals. The added bonus is you will be eating a much healthier diet. The more processed foods you avoid, the better.

Proteins, carbohydrates and fats

Buy these foods in their most natural form. They all get processed one way or another from some form of harvesting. Always check the label in case there is a risk of contamination.

Protein	Carbohydrates	Fats
• Beef • Turkey • Chicken • Pork (Ham, Bacon) • Eggs • Fish • Lamb	• Asparagus • Avocados • Black Beans • Broccoli • Brussels Sprouts • Cabbage • Carrots • Cauliflower • Cucumbers • Kidney Beans • Lettuce • Mushrooms • Onions • Peas • Peppers • Potato • Spinach	• Almonds • Brazil nuts • Blue Cheese • Brie Cheese • Cashews • Stilton Cheese • Soft Cheese

You might notice cheese included on the list of fats. Cheese is normally gluten free.

Liven up your meal

These condiments are safe to include with your meals:

- Butter
- Cinnamon
- Ginger
- Honey
- Paprika
- Parmesan
- Safflower oil
- Sage
- Salt
- Spices
- Tabasco sauce

This isn't a definitive list. There are many more you can eat, but these will help you get started.

Let's look at what you can drink.

6 drinks you can have today

Similar to food, always double check the labels on your drinks. You will be surprised what has been added to even the most basic of products.

1. Water. Obvious one, but water is safe to drink. Phew! You should watch out for flavoured waters as some of these can contain gluten.

If you are not a big fan of drinking plain water then why not make your own? Add some fresh cucumber, lemon, orange or lime to your water to inject flavour.

2. 100% fruit juices. Enjoy 100% fruit juices as they should be gluten free. Watch out for juices that come in cans or are dehydrated (powder) as they may have gluten added.

3. Tea. Tea comes from the camellia sinensis plant and is naturally gluten free. Be careful with herbal teas as they sometimes have barley added as a sweetener. You may even find 'pure' teas that have gluten added for flavour so always read the label.

4. Carbonated drinks. Most drinks like cola and lemonade are considered gluten free. But if you are super sensitive to gluten be careful with carbonated drinks. They have been known to cause reactions, which could be due to the certain additives containing trace amounts of gluten.

5. Drink coffee at home. Most coffee shops like Starbucks and Costa use gluten free beans but you cannot guarantee they will not be contaminated by gluten in the store. To reduce your risk make sure you advise the barista of your allergy. Play it safe and drink coffee you make at home. Most brands are gluten free.

6. Alcohol. Wine is naturally gluten free and should be fine for most people to drink. If you are extremely sensitive to gluten, proceed with caution. There is a chance that your wine could be contaminated with small traces of gluten during production from the use of fining agents and storage casks. Manufactures are not required to note trace amounts of gluten on wine labels. When in doubt call the manufacturer.

If you are a beer, ale, or lager drinker unfortunately most of these contain gluten. You will need to look for gluten free alternatives on the market for these types of drinks.

CHAPTER 5:

How to Cook Simple, Easy Gluten Free Meals

Day 2 Tips

Now it's time to turn those lists of gluten free foods into meals you can enjoy right now. The goal is to create gluten free meals with balance. Not only does this healthy approach give you the nutrients you need, it will leave you feeling fuller and more satisfied after your meals.

The 'recipe' is to add a Protein, a Carbohydrate, and a Fat together to create a meal. You can replace the Fat with another Carb if you are struggling for inspiration.

When determining portion sizes I always use the size of my hand clenched for Proteins and Carbs and then add as small an amount of Fat to my plate as possible.

Let's have a look at some examples.

Quick and easy meals you can prepare today

Day 1

Breakfast: smoked salmon and scrambled eggs on spinach

Lunch: cod, potato and peas

Dinner: turkey steaks, cauliflower and broccoli

Snacks: celery and peanut butter, orange

Day 2

Breakfast: bacon, eggs, mushrooms and baked beans

Lunch: jacket potato and cottage cheese

Dinner: sirloin steak, sweet potato and mushrooms

Snacks: banana, handful of raisins and nuts

Meals you can create with gluten free alternatives

Now let's dive into detail regarding gluten free alternatives, like gluten free bread and pasta. I've also included some simple meals you can create with these products.

1. **Gluten free bread.** Once you have some gluten free bread it opens your world up to most of the recipes you would have eaten before. You can now have bacon sandwiches, beef burgers, and ham and cheese sandwiches.

2. **Gluten free pasta.** Gluten free pasta helps round out some of your meals. You might want to get some gluten free cooking sauces to add to them. My favourite is diced chicken with pasta and cream cheese. Mix cream cheese into the pasta to make a great gluten free sauce.

3. **Gluten free breadcrumbs.** You can liven up any meats on your protein list with breadcrumbs. Coat your fish in breadcrumbs and have fish and chips. Add them to chicken or turkey breasts to create the breaded versions. Just make sure they are certified gluten free!

4. **Gluten free noodles.** Dice some chicken, chop up some vegetables and you have yourself a stir fry. Make sure you buy a gluten free sauce to go with as most stir fry sauces contain gluten.

4 snacks you can take on the move

It is important to have snacks handy when you go out. You do not want to be caught unprepared with nothing safe to eat. Here are four easy-to-prepare ideas to get you started.

1. **Fruit.** The easiest to prepare of all! Ensure you keep a supply of fruit handy. You can take fruit anywhere with you. Not only is it healthy, it will give you a quick hunger fix.

2. **Lettuce wraps.** This snack is best eaten at home unless you have a refrigerated bag. Why not wrap your meats and fillings in lettuce to make a healthy gluten free sandwich? My favourite is the tuna lettuce wrap.

3. **Rice cakes.** Most plain rice cakes are gluten free. They make a great go-to product when you need a snack. The combinations you can create with toppings are endless. Eat them on their own or with cottage cheese or peanut butter. You can also eat them with any type of fruit.

4. **Mixed nuts and dried fruits.** Carry a bag of mixed nuts and dried fruits with you when you go out. You don't need to worry about keeping them refrigerated.

CHAPTER 6:

Shopping for Gluten Free Products

You now know what you are going to be eating for the next couple of days. You even have enough ideas to keep you going for a few weeks. Now it's time to buy everything you need to make your meals.

Think back to the Olympian mindset and preparation. It is key that you plan your meals, write a shopping list and allow enough time for your shopping trip. Let's look at why this helps.

1. Plan your meals. Make sure you don't get overwhelmed by planning out your meals. You should think about the following:

- Shop in one go. It takes a lot of energy trying to decide what to eat on the spot. Why not do it in one sitting and plan for the week? Then go get what you need from the market.

- Don't shop when hungry. Trying to decide what to eat when you are hungry is the worst thing you can do. You are more likely to cheat and give in to temptation or rush and not take precautions.

- Get yourself a meal planner for your fridge. If it's visible you are more likely to stick to it.

- Don't forget to plan your snacks for each day. You want to be prepared when hunger strikes. This is even more important when you are out and about all day.

2. Write a shopping list. Transfer your meal plan onto a shopping list. You want to know exactly what you are looking for when you head to the supermarket.

3. Allow enough time. This is your first gluten free shopping trip so it is going to take you a while. It is important that you get the right products and not buy anything with gluten in it. This can be an easy mistake to make. You need to read the label of every product you pick up, even if you bought it before. Suppliers change their recipes all the time. The one time you don't check the label, you will wake up the following day regretting it.

Allow enough time so that you don't feel rushed and can read every label.

Understanding food labels

The majority of the food you purchase using our foods lists will be naturally gluten free. But you need to know if each item is safe to purchase or not. The easiest and quickest way to tell if something has gluten in it is by reading the label.

Laws in the UK and EU have improved over the last 10 years which makes it much easier to identify if your product is gluten free or not. Let's see what you should be looking for on the back of your product. There are 4 different situations you will be faced with.

1. Clearly labelled 'gluten free.'

If a product is gluten free, then 'gluten free' will normally be displayed on the front of the packaging. Companies like to highlight the benefits of purchasing gluten free products. You might find a product is gluten free even if it isn't labelled as such on the front, as it is not a legal requirement to do so.

When in doubt move to the back of the packaging and look for dietary information or ingredients.

The term gluten free can only be used on foods that contain 20 parts per million (ppm) or less of gluten. This should be safe for anyone that is not super-sensitive.

2. Contains 'gluten.'

At the other end of the spectrum, it is UK and EU Law to state the ingredients on the label. These are the ingredients you should be looking out for:

- wheat

- rye

- barley

- oats

- spelt

- khorasan wheat (commercially known as Kamut®).

If a product contains an allergen then it will normally be in **bold**. For example, on the back of the packaging it will say:

- Contains Wheat

- Contains Rye

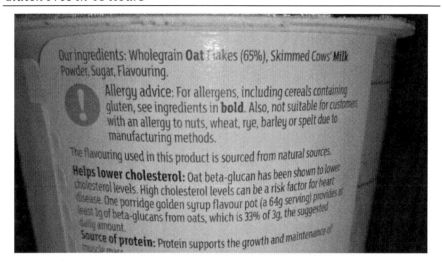

You MUST avoid products containing these statements.

3. May contain traces of gluten.

This is where we start getting away from the clear cut statements on packaging. This is the manufacturers 'get out of jail free' card. They can't guarantee that it hasn't been contaminated either during manufacture or preparation stage.

Eat products labelled this way at your own risk. You can also contact the manufacturer directly if you would like further information about product safety.

4. Not suitable for people with coeliac disease/a wheat allergy due to manufacturing methods.

This phrase is exactly the same as 'may contain traces of gluten' and you will find it worded in different ways. Other alternates are:

- made on a line handling wheat

- made in factory also handling wheat

This means the product could have been contaminated from

their processing machinery as it could have previously handled gluten products. Same as above, eat these products at your own risk or contact the manufacturer first.

4 things to consider about the 'Free From' section

In the UK the majority of supermarkets have a section called the 'Free From' section. This can be a great place to buy products that are gluten free. There are a few things you have to watch out for, though.

1. Not everything is gluten free. The majority of this section is gluten free but some product lines are just 'free' from general allergens. Always double check the label before you buy. You will find products that are dairy, soya and nut free here too.

2. Price. Unfortunately due to all the hype around gluten free diets the market has been flooded with new gluten free products. This is obviously not a bad thing from a choice perspective but it comes at a cost. You could end up spending 4 times the amount on gluten free products in the Free From section as compared to elsewhere in the store. Manufacturers have jumped on the bandwagon to get their piece of the gluten free pie.

Tip: Shop for your supermarket's own Free From branded products. They will be a lot cheaper than the mainstream branded products.

3. Quality. How do you make something gluten free? You have to substitute gluten with something and in most cases gluten is substituted with fat and sugar. Keep an eye on the nutritional values of what you buy from the Free From section. When it comes to snack bars and treats you will be eating more calories than your standard chocolate bar.

4. Shop for essentials. There are a few items to watch for as we have discussed but there are some products you will just have to buy from the Free From aisle:

- Pasta

- Bread and cakes

- Flour

- The occasional treat

Keep it simple and use products from this section as part of your go-forward diet for the time being.

CHAPTER 7:

Avoid 'Beginner Mistakes' in the First 48 Hours

Well done. You have made it so far, you are well on your way to a gluten free life.

It wasn't as hard as you first thought it was going to be, was it?

You have followed each step carefully. Then it hits you. You feel like you have been struck with a full-on body flu. Stomach cramps and diarrhea follow.

You have been so careful, right? You haven't eaten anything with gluten in it.

Or have you?

What has just happened to you is the term 'glutened'. You have ingested or come into contact with something containing gluten.

What could it have been? How could this have happened? Let's discuss what can go wrong in your first 48 hours.

6 products that surprisingly contain gluten

Watch out for these and other products you may not suspect contain gluten. There might be something you just take for granted is gluten free—but it's not.

1. **Soy sauce**. Wheat is perhaps the last thing you associate with soy sauce, but it is a key part of the manufacturing process. Soy sauce is made with fermented wheat. If you are eating out then make sure you bring your own gluten

free soy sauce.

2. **Gravy and oxo cubes.** Different types of gravies and stocks are made with flour. They can also contain barley in the flavourings.

3. **French fries and chips.** Naturally gluten free, I can understand why you might think chips and fries are safe. They are just chopped up potato right?

Wrong! There are so many different ways they can get contaminated. Some have flour added to them to make them crispier. They could be fried in a chip fryer that has been contaminated. Many chip shops will reuse oil and this could contaminate the chips if it had battered products in it previously.

4. **Oats.** There is a bit of conflicting information about oats. Oats contain avenin, which is a protein similar to gluten. According to Coeliac UK the UK charity for coeliac disease, most people with coeliac disease can eat avenin safely.

There are a few cases of people that are really sensitive having a reaction to pure oats so be aware that you could still have a reaction. If you can tolerate oats then I would definitely keep them as part of your diet. They are a good source of fiber.

Are all oats safe? No, in fact there are many brands that are not gluten free. This is usually because they are processed in the same place as barley, wheat or rye. Always ensure you buy gluten free pure oats.

5. **Condiments**. This can be a tricky one and I would always read the label when buying condiments. If you are eating out then try and avoid anything with sauce. Gluten is used as a stabiliser and thickener in a lot of condiments.

Gluten can lurk in:

- Ketchup

- Mustard

- Pasta sauce

- Tomato paste

- Marinades

- Salad dressings

- Worcester sauce

6. Medication. Be wary of gluten in medication if you're still feeling ill and have a clean diet. Gluten can be used in medications as a binder which aids digestion for those without gluten sensitivities.

It can be tough to identify if your medication is safe as they won't always state on the packaging if it is gluten free because it might only contain trace amounts. You will have to sift through the ingredients to find anything that might suggest gluten. If in doubt then you should always call the manufacturer.

5 ways to recover quickly when you have been glutened

So you have made a mistake or you have given into temptation. Either way, it is important that you get straight back on track. You want to recover as quickly as possible. Here are 6 ways that you can do just that.

1. Stop, drop and rest. Remember earlier I said your immune system was waging war on gluten? Well this war can take it out of you. If you don't rest up it will take longer to recover. I know this might be hard especially if you live a busy life but the quicker you rest the quicker you will be back to your best.

Don't feel like you have to fight through it. You won't win any medals. If you can jump straight into bed, please do. Toughing it out could end up putting you out of commission for days.

2. **Drink plenty of water**. Water flushes out excess fluids and toxins making it quicker to flush gluten out of your system.

- Add lemon to your water as it will support your liver and kidneys. It will help them naturally remove toxins from your body.

- Add ginger to your water as it has natural anti-inflammatory properties. It will help your stomach when it becomes bloated.

Pour boiling water over ginger, let steep for about 5 minutes then add lemon juice.

3. **Take digestive enzymes**. Digestive enzymes help your body break down food in your stomach. They are a very debatable method to speed up the healing process. It has been said that digestive enzymes will help break down gluten in your stomach, helping you digest and remove it from your body more quickly.

That being said, it works for some people and others see no effect. Advocates could be experiencing a placebo effect, but either way it has benefitted some.

4. **Take charcoal tablets**. I first discovered this as a cure for travel sickness but charcoal tablets have other benefits too. The reason they help travel sickness is because they reduce bloating and settle your stomach. Charcoal tablets will help you tolerate the symptoms you get from being glutened. Watch out though as charcoal can absorb medications and make them ineffective.

5. Eat bone broth. Eating bone broth is a favourite amongst the coeliac community. Bone broth promotes healthy digestion because of nutrients absorbed by the bones. Get yourself some bone broth from Amazon for an instant fix but you can also make it yourself. There are some pre-made bone broths that contain gluten so be careful when ordering.

It is best to make bone broth yourself. Invest in a slow cooker and cook vegetables, bones and water for 12 hours.

Let's recap. When you are glutened get into bed with your favourite lemon and ginger water and eat nothing but bone broth. You will be feeling better in no time.

What to do if you still feel sick

You have gone gluten free for a few months now. You haven't cheated and have been trying really hard. So why do you still feel the same? Why have your symptoms not improved?

Do you continue to suffer with abdominal pain, bloating, flatulence, diarrhea and nausea? It may not be anything you are doing wrong. It might be you are suffering from something else.

If you suffered from coeliac for quite a while then you have sustained quite a bit of damage to your gut. It can take quite a while to heal. Coeliac has left your gut weak and at this point you could be reacting to something else.

You could be lactose intolerant

I know a lot of people that have given up gluten and dairy because their stomach struggles with both. These two conditions are quite regularly linked together, due to the gut damage.

If you suspect that dairy is causing trouble then remove it from your diet. Try and remove it for 30 days to see if it makes any real difference. Some people go dairy free then start adding dairy back into their diet later down the line. Others stay dairy free for life. It all depends on your body.

If you want to try both, consider a Paleo diet. Paleo is the closest regime that fits being gluten free and dairy free.

You are on a journey

Remember you are only just starting your journey. Don't beat yourself up when you make a mistake. You will learn and you will adapt. It WILL get easier as time passes.

Even seasoned coeliacs still make mistakes. They get lazy. They forget to read labels.

You will make mistakes.

It is important you get back on the horse and carry on. Remember, your health is at stake right?

SUMMARY

How to go Gluten Free in 10 Steps

That brings us to the end of the book. We have taken you through your first 48 hours of going gluten free. Step by step.

Just follow this plan and you will be well on your way to a gluten free life. Get started today. Let's recap each step.

1. Understand your condition. You can't go gluten free until you have been diagnosed. How do you know what changes you need to make when you don't understand your condition? **Get diagnosed** *before* **you start.**

2. You know why it is important to remove gluten FAST! Do you really want to live with constant pain? If you don't take action today you increase your risk of life threatening diseases like cancer. You could end up pooping through a bag for the rest of your life.

3. Adopt the 'preparation' mindset. You need to plan and prepare relentlessly. Plan your meals, your trips out, and your supermarket shopping for starters. If you get caught unprepared then you will get glutened.

Use our cheat sheet at **www.glutify.co.uk/gluten-free-cheatsheet** as your starter plan.

4. Clear out your system and kitchen. Flush out gluten by drinking plenty of water and eating plenty of vegetables. Most importantly, do not cheat! You want to remove anything that might contaminate your food in the future.

- Give away. Give away your condiments in jars, baking ingredients, baked goods, pasta, noodles, cereal, processed meat, fish, poultry and canned products.

- Replace. Replace your toaster, cookware and utensils, grill, and don't forget the colander!
- **Clean.** Clean your oven, fridge, grill, food preparation surfaces and your dining table.

Day 1

5. **Follow these segregation rules.**

- Label everything—make sure you don't pick up the wrong product.
- Segregate your cupboards and fridge—don't let gluten sneak in.
- Buy condiments in plastic squeeze bottles—prevent spoon contamination.
- Wash up separately—gluten can hide in your sponges and towels too.
- Prepare gluten free meals first—you can easily make a mistake when multi-tasking.

6. **You know the basics of what you CAN eat and drink.** Try to eat foods in their most natural form and use the list of basic food items you can eat. Then mix and match them to create meals. Don't try to over-complicate your meals until you get the basics right.

Protein + Carbohydrate + Fat (or another Carb) = Meal. Keep it simple!

Stick to simple drinks like water and 100% fruit juices.

Day 2

7. **You know how to prepare some quick and easy gluten free meals.** You have a few meals to get you started. You can

also get some gluten free bread, pasta and noodles and make your favourite recipes using our food guide. Remember to always carry fruit, nuts and rice cakes with you when on the move too.

8. You know how to prepare for your first supermarket trip. Plan out your meals, write out a shopping list and ensure you leave enough time for shopping.

9. You know how to check if something is gluten free.

- Always read the label.
- Gluten free doesn't always stay gluten free—read each label even if you bought it previously.
- Watch out for products made using unsafe manufacturing processes. Eat at your own risk.

10. You know how to avoid common beginner mistakes. If you do make a mistake, stop immediately and rest, drink plenty of water, take a charcoal tablet and finish it off with a hit of bone broth.

Go gluten free in 48 hours

I know it might feel overwhelming. There is a lot to take in. That is why I have broken everything down into small steps.

You have the plan. All you need to do is take action. One step at a time.

You will get results.

Tom
Glutify.co.uk

Thank you

I just want to say thank you for purchasing and reading this guide. You could have chosen a different book but you chose mine. I hope it helped you the same way it has helped others.

If you liked this guide then I need your help! I would really appreciate it if you left a review on Amazon. Your feedback will help me create books that help you reach your goals.

Resources

Cheat Sheet - www.glutify.co.uk/gluten-free-cheatsheet

Coeliac Disease: Do I Have It? How To Understand Your Symptoms, Condition and Get Diagnosed. FAST! - www.glutify.co.uk/understanding-your-condition

Sign up at www.glutify.co.uk for updates

Printed in Great Britain
by Amazon